Yoga for Beginners

Yoga for Beginners

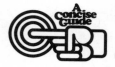

by Alice K. Turner

photographs by Meryl Joseph

FRANKLIN WATTS, INC. • NEW YORK

Library of Congress Cataloging in Publication Data

Turner, Alice K.
    Yoga for beginners.

    (A Concise guide)
    SUMMARY: An introduction to yoga with instructions
for simple exercises.
    1. Yoga–Juvenile literature. [1. Yoga]
I. Joseph, Meryl, illus. II. Title.
RA781.7.T87   613.7   73-5712
ISBN 0-531-02643-4
ISBN 0-531-02412-1 (pbk)
Copyright © 1973 by Alice K. Turner
Printed in the United States
5 4 3 2 1

Contents

Yoga for Beginners

*Why
Study
Yoga?*

We Americans think about exercise a great deal, even if we
don't do much about it. Magazines publish fitness programs.
People get up early in the morning to do their "jerks" — or at
least they talk about how they *should* be getting up early. Some
people go to exercise classes, some play tennis or golf, some jog
or swim. Look in your local bookstore and you'll find numerous
books and pamphlets on exercise and fitness regimes. And in
most areas, you'll find at least one half-hour television program
devoted to physical exercise.

Undoubtedly, our concern with fitness is a good thing. Nevertheless, it's a fact that most Americans are not particularly fit —
in other words, they have good reason to be concerned. Older
people are often very inactive, which soon results in the "spare
tires" around their middles and the generally soft look that
comes from loss of muscle tone. Young people are usually far
more active. Small children prefer running to walking; they
climb trees, wrestle, play strenuous games, and in general manage to wear themselves out each day. (They wear out their
mothers too!) But by the time they reach their teens, often all
this energy just seems to drain away.

1

Schools don't help much. The typical pattern in junior high and high school is an intense athletic program for those students (mostly boys) who have made one of the school teams, and almost nothing for the others. For nonathletes who drive or are driven to school, exercise comes mostly in short occasional bursts — a night of strenuous dancing here, a long walk there, a skiing weekend once a year, an impromptu game of volleyball. The natural inertia that plagues us, now that we no longer have to hunt down or hoe down tonight's dinner, has begun to set in. Before much time has passed, the trim teenager is putting on that middle-aged spread that in many cases is caused less by overeating than by simple lack of exercise.

A regular pattern of exercise is almost essential to the maintenance of continuing good health and good looks, and the very best time to get into this pattern is the teens. (It's true that newspapers are always publishing birthday stories about hale old geezers who boast that they never exercised a day in their lives — but these stories should be taken with an ounce or so of salt.) Think about it — if you start the habit of exercising in your teens, when most likely your body is in pretty good shape, you'll never have to do any *remedial* exercise. That is, you'll never have to pull the old body out of the flabby slump it's gotten into. It does make sense to start now.

As should be clear from the title of this book, the exercise recommended here is yoga, or, to be specific, *hatha-yoga. Hatha-yoga* is the study of physical discipline through the practice of learned techniques involving *asanas,* or poses, and breathing. This *hatha-yoga,* or physical yoga, is a very old discipline that evolved in India over a thousand years ago. It is what we Westerners think of when we use the word "yoga." Actually the word means "discipline" (the word "yoke" in the sense of a yoke for oxen comes from the same root), and *hatha-yoga* is only one of a number of yogic disciplines, often religious or mystical, taught in India.

Hatha-yoga can be studied without any religious overtones, however, and undoubtedly most people who make it part of their lives approach it from a physical rather than a spiritual angle. This is true in India also. There has been a great interest in Eastern religion here in the last decade, and many of the yoga centers in the United States do have a religious affiliation. Nevertheless, interest in yoga is often — in fact, usually — quite secular. Westerners have been interested in it for a long time. Martha Graham and other pioneers of modern dance revolutionized the physical approach to dance, and in doing so, they borrowed many techniques from yoga.

Advanced *hatha-yoga* requires a good deal of strength and can involve some truly awesome feats of body control. But great strength is not needed for the exercises described in this book. These have been taught to beginners in essentially the same pattern for hundreds of years, and the only requirements for learning them are patience and willingness. Even people with some disability or physical handicap can study yoga. If you think, however, that this makes yoga babyish or too simple a discipline, reserve judgment until you've tried it.

Why is yoga better for you than other programs of physical exercise? Well, it's probably better to avoid comparatives like "better," but yoga does offer certain advantages. To begin with, even the beginner's routine offers *complete* exercise, stretching and toning all parts of the body, literally from the toes to the top of the head!

Second, because it depends on the slow mastery of body disciplines and avoids strenuous activity, it's less tiring and really less boring than most physical programs. One can dread an energetic series of sitting-up exercises, but no one dreads yoga; it's soothing as well as invigorating.

Third, it's absolutely noncompetitive, as you are working only with your own body. Some classes, in fact, ask beginners to keep their eyes closed till they have recovered from their

3

self-consciousness and stopped trying to do better than other people in the class.

Fourth, yoga is equally effective for boys and girls. In fact, because girls are usually more supple, they tend to be better at it, at least at first.

Fifth, because yoga teaches awareness of how the body moves and operates, persons studying it often begin to treat their bodies better, learning new eating and drinking habits. No one who really gets into breathing is going to continue smoking cigarettes.

And sixth, you can do yoga by yourself. It's true that studying with a teacher, at least for a while, is essential if you are going to get serious about yoga, but eventually everyone works by himself. In the long run, this is a tremendous advantage because it frees you from dependence on any class or person.

And lastly, yoga is fun. It gets your blood running, it does wonders for your complexion, it improves your posture and your bendability and teaches you how to breathe properly. Also you learn to stand on your head, to twist yourself into exotic shapes, and to look at things from a very different point of view. Sharing it with your friends can be fun, but it's also fun to do all by yourself.

Work hard, but enjoy it!

Before You Start

It's a good idea to find one special private place to perform your daily routine. Your bedroom is a good choice, if you can be sure you won't be interrupted while you're concentrating. If you share a bedroom, you can either ask for half an hour of privacy each day or else get your brother or sister to join in for a team effort. In either case, no spectators, please!

The time of day for your yoga session is up to you. In India, it's thought to be most beneficial first thing in the morning, before breakfast. That's often such a busy time of day, however, what with getting ready for school and deciding what to wear and waiting your turn in the bathroom, that it's often better to postpone your session until later. After school is a good time. Or just before you start your homework — you'll feel so refreshed you'll get through it in half the time. Or just before bed. Any time is okay except for just after a meal. You don't have to do it at exactly the same time each day, but it's easier if you get into a routine.

You need flexible clothing, that is, no tight jeans, belts, or anything else to encumber you. On the other hand, loose pajamas or shirts may bunch up awkwardly around you. In general, the less you wear the better. Underwear is good, or perhaps a bathing suit, or shorts and a t-shirt, or a leotard. No shoes, of course, though socks are fine if your feet are cold. If your hair is long, secure it with a rubber band or a barrette.

You'll also need a towel or towel-sized mat. This is to keep you clean (so keep *it* clean) and to cushion you slightly from the hard floor. (You don't have to actually lie on the floor; a rug is fine, so long as the pile isn't deep and it won't slip.)

Now you're ready to begin. But don't rush into it. Slow and steady always wins in yoga. Don't watch the clock either (if you have only a limited amount of time, set the alarm or a kitchen timer so that you won't keep glancing up at the clock and breaking your concentration). New exercises naturally take longer to do properly than familiar ones, so give yourself plenty of time in the beginning.

As you attempt each *asana*, you should go about it methodically. You won't perform it perfectly the first day or even the first week. Nobody expects you to, so relax.

First, concentrate carefully on perfecting the right mechanical technique, getting each step down by heart so you don't have to think about it.

Second, relax. Be as economical with your muscles as you can, using only the ones that are essential to the movement you are performing. This usually takes more time than the first step. Watch your face — it tends to tense up.

Third, adjust your breathing. Don't forget that *hatha-yoga* involves physical postures *and breathing*. Your breathing must be smooth, even, and controlled. Beginners almost always tend to hold their breath while doing difficult movements. The directions for each *asana* include breathing instructions, or if they don't, you assume that your breathing should be completely regular. More about breathing later.

Fourth, smooth your performance down to a continuous, steady movement, nothing jerky, hasty, or delayed. Your body should operate in one fluid, oiled movement, relaxed and totally controlled. As your concentration improves, your movements will become easier, and as your movements become easier, your concentration will improve.

6

Stre-e-e-e-e-tch Yourself!

Lie down on your back on your towel with your legs slightly apart and your hands alongside your body, palms up and fingers half-closed. In other words, get as comfortable as you possibly can, making sure your neck muscles are not tense.

Now, concentrate on the toes of your left foot. Tense them as hard as you can while leaving all the rest of your muscles relaxed. Tense your whole left foot. Now slowly tense your right toes and your right foot.

Next tense your left leg working upward slowly from the ankle to the buttock. Do the same with your right leg.

Beginning with the fingers, slowly tense your left arm up to the shoulder. Now your right arm.

Pull in your stomach and tense your torso, feeling the tightening of the chest muscles.

Tense your neck and pull your chin in hard.

Scrunch up your face muscles as tightly as you can — still remembering to breathe evenly — till you feel that every inch of your body from your scalp to your toenails is drawn tightly.

Now begin to let go, starting with your head and face muscles, and continuing on down the way you came, as slowly and smoothly as you can. When you have relaxed the last toe, simply lie there, breathing in and out for a few moments.

7

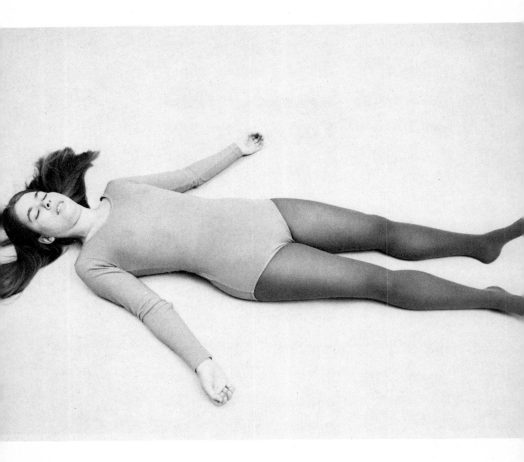

*Learn to tense and
relax each muscle.*

Don't you feel good? Now you are really relaxed, far more
than when you first lay down. What's more, this simple exercise
acquaints you with your body, helping you to isolate the muscles that control each part. Begin and end your session this way.
Also use this as a simple technique for relaxing when you feel
yourself getting tired and tense. Try it in bed, too, as a sleep
inducer.

Salute
to the
Sun

Traditionally, Hindu yogis (a yogi is one who practices yoga) perform the Salute to the Sun at dawn, facing the east as the sun rises. As they greet the new day, they reacquaint themselves with their own bodies, for the Salute to the Sun is splendidly complete, stretching the spine and the muscles, deepening the breathing. It's a fine way to get the day going, but it's equally useful if you do it later on.

There are twelve movements to the complete Salute, the last six being the first six in reverse. It will take you a while to get to the point where you can run through all twelve movements evenly, keeping your breathing regular. (Though breathing is always important, emphasis is placed on it here, for the Salute is considered to be an ideal combination of stretching and breathing.) Eventually you'll fall into the right rhythm, and the whole sequence should take about twenty seconds.

1. Stand comfortably erect, feet together, hands folded in a prayer position at your chest. Breathe out slowly.

2. Raise your arms and head slowly, stretching backward and upward and breathing in.

3. Bend forward and place your hands on the floor, or as

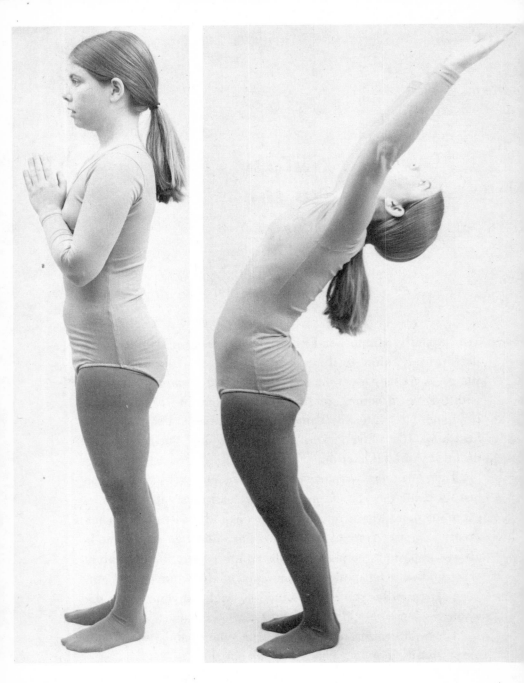

Left: the prayer position.
Right: stretch up and back.

10

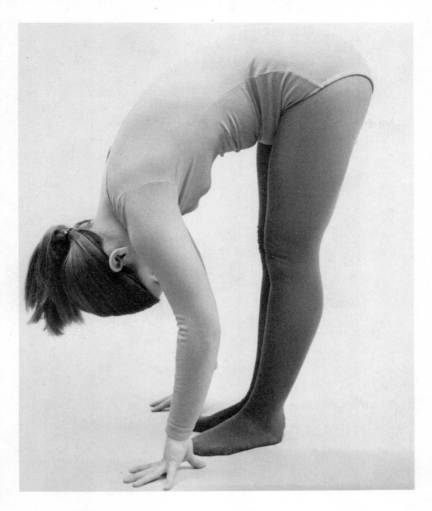

Try to touch your head to your knees.

close to it as you can manage. Bring your head as close as possible to your knees. As you continue to breathe out evenly,
stretch downward and closer to your knees. Bend your knees
slightly if you must. After a week or so of doing this exercise
regularly, your spine will already be more flexible.

4. Take your weight upon your hands. Stretch your right
leg backward in a big step, gripping the floor with your right
toes and keeping your left foot firmly on the floor between your
hands. Inhale as you do this.

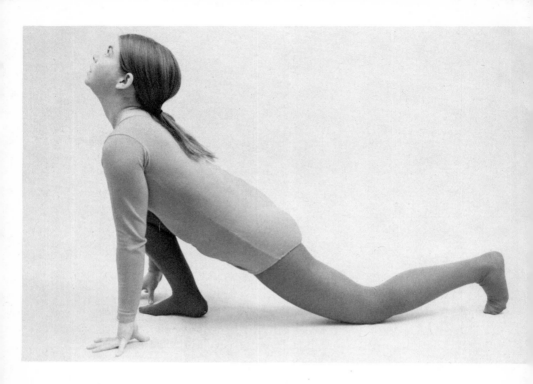

One leg goes back . . .
. . . then the other.

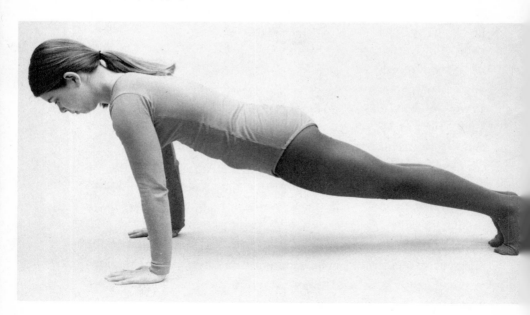

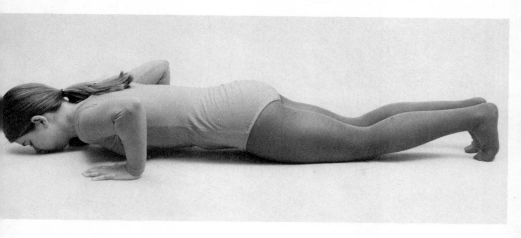

Lower yourself gently to the floor.

5. Exhale. Then stretch your left leg backward to meet the right, keeping your body in a straight line from head to heels. Inhale as you do this.

6. Exhale, lowering your body to the floor as though you were coming down from a push-up, but keeping your buttocks slightly raised so that finally you touch the floor with only eight parts of your body — your two feet (actually, it's your ten toes, but why quibble?), two knees, chest, two hands, and forehead. It's considered best to hold the head in such a way that *only* the forehead touches, the nose being kept off the floor.

7. Inhale, and bend backward as far as you can, pointing your toes and looking up. By itself, this is called the Cobra Pose. Hold it, stretching backward and breathing in and out a few times comfortably.

8. Exhale, lifting the buttocks up in the air. Ideally, the hands and feet should now be flat on the floor, but few beginners can manage to keep their heels down. So stay in this pose (it's called the Dog Pose) a few moments, breathing in and out, and alternately pushing your right and left heels toward the floor. This will gradually stretch your ligaments, though it will make them sore at first. Don't worry; the soreness will pass. Keep your head down during the Dog Pose.

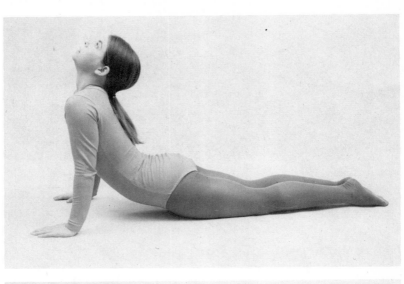

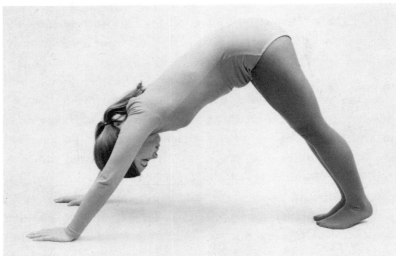

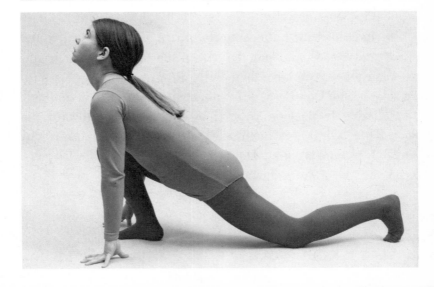

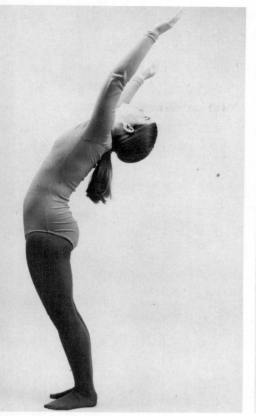
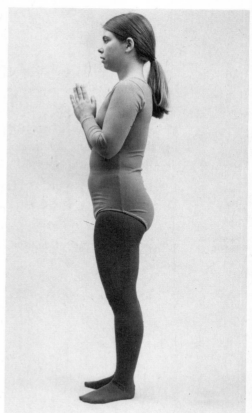

Up and back again ... and finish in a prayer pose.

9. Bring your right leg forward, placing it between your hands. Inhale as you do it.

10. Exhale, bring the left leg forward. Inhale, pressing the head to the knees.

11. Straighten up slowly, inhaling, and raise the arms overhead, bending backward.

12. Exhale, coming back to the prayer position. Rest a few moments, breathing in and out.

Top: the Cobra position.
Center: the Dog position.
Bottom: one leg comes forward, then the other.

15

In your first few sessions, it might be a good idea for you to concentrate on this one essential exercise rather than going on to anything else. If you decide to do this, which would show patience and discipline truly worthy of a yogi, you might follow up these sessions by doing the preliminary steps to the Headstand (see page 43). By the time you've got the Salute down to the point where you're ready to tackle something new, you'll be ready for the Headstand proper.

The Salute to the Sun should always be the first exercise you do after stretching because it gets your body ready for things to come.

The Shoulder Stand and the Plow

This double *asana* is considered to be, together with the Salute to the Sun, the most basic and important of yogic exercises. Muscles in your stomach, spine, neck, and legs all come into play, and any inverted position is considered to activate the circulation — which is good for your skin. If for any reason you should have to limit the time for yoga, you can get a fairly complete workout with just the Salute to the Sun and this one.

1. Lie flat on your back on your towel with your hands palms down near your thighs. Keeping your knees straight and your feet close together but not pointed (you want to keep your calves and thighs relaxed, letting your stomach muscles do the work), raise your legs slowly up to a vertical position. *Don't hold your breath;* keep breathing regularly and calmly.

2. Without breaking your rhythm, let your body follow your legs up into the air. Bend your arms at the elbows and let your hands support your back. Straighten your body as much as possible, tightening your buttocks to do so. Your chin will be tucked into your chest and the nape of your neck will be flat against the floor. Breathe in and out evenly and enjoy this novel postion.

3. Now, very slowly, lower your right leg to the floor — or as close to the floor as you can get — behind your head.

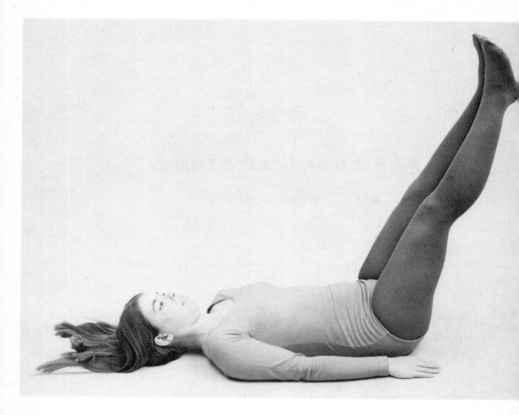

Keep your knees straight.

Slowly bring it up again and do the same with your left leg. Keep breathing evenly and try to avoid any scissors motion with your legs.

4. Now let both legs together go to the floor behind your head. Let them fall of their own weight, but slowly. Don't worry if your toes won't reach the floor. After just a few regular sessions they'll get there with no effort at all on your part. As you are doing this, straighten your arms out again, palms to the floor, to help you balance. You are now in the Plow Pose and you should stay there for a few moments, breathing regularly and keeping your knees straight. If you want to contemplate your navel, you have a fine view!

18

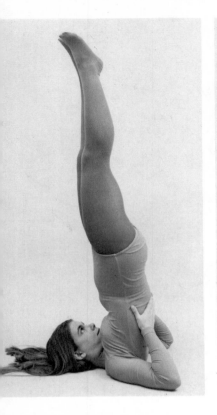
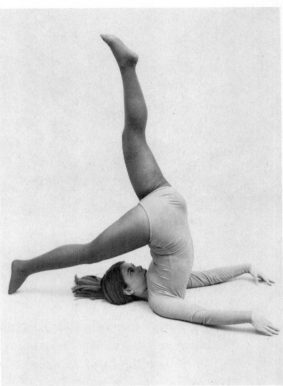

Top left: the Shoulder Stand;
right: lower one leg gently to the floor.
Bottom: the Plow.

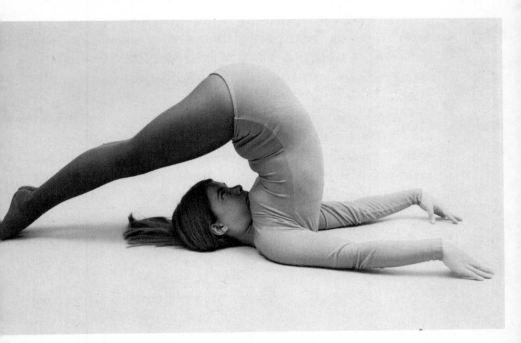

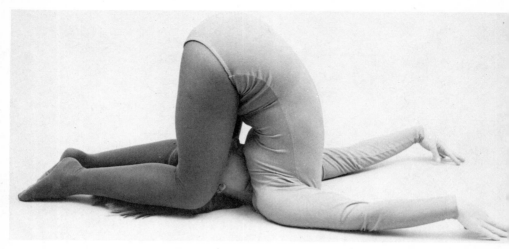

Knees to the ears.

5. Bend your knees and bring them down to your ears. Hold this pose for a few breaths.

6. As you slowly straighten your legs again, begin to uncurl. Imagine that you are uncurling your spine one joint at a time, controlling the speed of your movement with great care till you are again flat on your back with your legs in the air.

7. Without breaking rhythm, begin to lower your legs slowly to the floor. Don't let them fall. In fact, you should hold them motionless for a moment at about two inches from the floor before you finally bring them down.

8. Relax, breathing softly, for a few moments. You'll be grateful for the rest, particularly in the beginning, as this sequence is a tough one. You'll find, however, that it gets easier rapidly as your spine becomes more flexible and your stomach muscles harder.

An extra advantage to the Plow Pose is that, quite inevitably, it gets you thinking about the shape you're in. If you've somehow managed to put on a few extra pounds around your middle, you're going to be made very aware of that fact. This may encourage you to take them off right away. The beauty of the Plow Pose is that, because it exercises those very stomach muscles, it actually helps you to do just that.

The Fish

It's a good idea to do the Fish right after the Shoulder-Stand-Plow because it bends the spine in the opposite direction. The Fish is also marvellous exercise for your thighs and buttocks, so people with problems in those areas should concentrate on this one.

1. Sit squarely on your heels. Now, keeping your knees together, move your feet apart so that you're actually sitting *between* your heels. This is usually easier for girls than boys, but with practice anyone can do it. Tuck your toes under your buttocks and put your hands on your heels. Keep those knees together all during the exercise — it won't be easy.

2. Lean your body back and slightly to the right, leaning your right elbow on the floor, then adjusting your body so that you're leaning on both elbows.

3. Lean your head backward as far as you can, arching your chest and hollowing your back.

4. Fold your hands on your chest and rest your head on the floor. Arch your body, still keeping your knees together and your buttocks firmly on the floor. Hold this postition for about ten breaths.

5. Clasp your heels again and come up to your elbows. Reverse the procedure you used in getting down to the floor; that is, shift your body so that you return to a sitting position by way of one elbow.

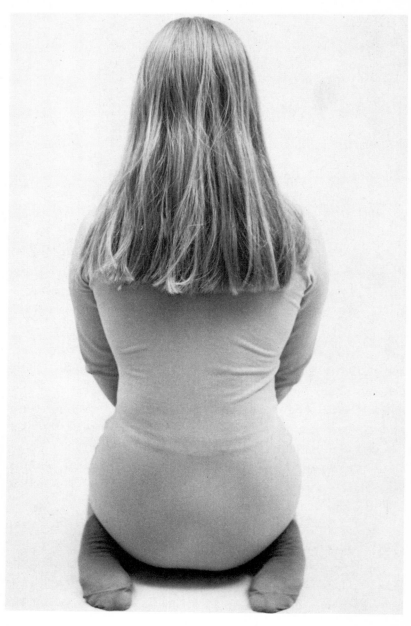

Knees together as you sit between your feet.

Top: lean first on one elbow, then on both.
Center: the Fish.
Bottom: rest your head on your knees.

22

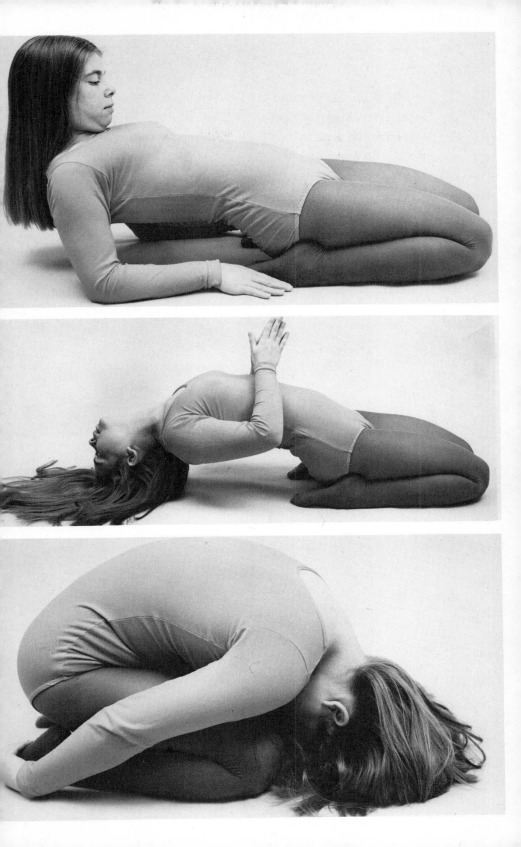

6. Without breaking your rhythm, bend forward until your head is touching your knees, or is as close to them as you can get comfortably. Rest in this position for a few moments before returning to a sitting position.

The Forward Bend

This exercise will remind you of sit-ups and other phys-ed standbys. There's a big difference, however. In yoga every movement must be slow, regular, and not at all sudden or jerky; and you must keep your breathing calm and smooth.

There are several variations on the Forward Bend. Because they are such good stretching and stomach-tightening exercises, you may want to do them all if you have time.

1. Lie flat on your back with your arms stretched out behind your head. Link your thumbs together and keep your body relaxed.

2. Raise your arms to the vertical while your body remains motionless. Then let them slowly drop toward your thighs while your head and shoulders rise from the floor. Keep your back firmly on the floor and focus your eyes on your fingers.

3. As your fingers reach your thighs, unlink them and push them lightly along your legs toward your feet, letting the body follow — first it is raised to a sitting position, and then it begins to lean forward. Bring your forehead down as close to your knees as possible. Grasp your big toes with your hands, if you can reach them, or your ankles if you can't. You should try to

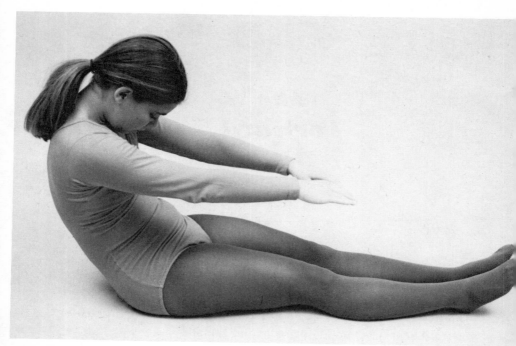

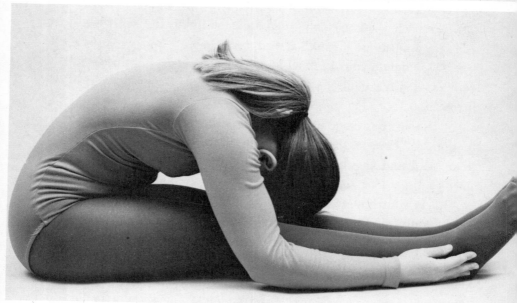

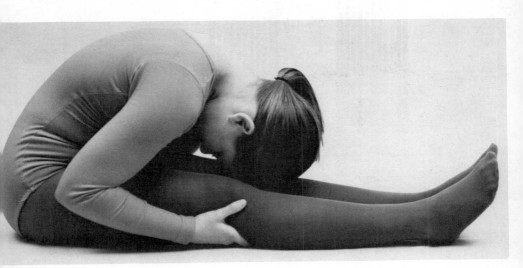

Grip your knees and pull your head down.

keep your knees locked and your legs straight, but if you simply can't do that, bend them a little. Practice will make perfect. Incidentally, if you find that your stomach muscles aren't strong enough to raise your body from the floor at first, try hooking your toes under a sofa or another heavy piece of furniture. Breathe in as your body rises from the floor, and breathe out as you lower your head to your knees.

4. Slowly return to your starting position, uncurling your spine one joint at a time, starting with the base. Your hands should remain on your thighs till almost all of your back is on the floor.

Variation 1. Instead of trying to catch your big toes, grasp your knees with your thumbs over your kneecaps and the other fingers under the knee and the elbows close to the thighs. Push your arms back toward your body at the same time that you try

Top: come up slowly from the floor.
Bottom: head to knees, hands stretched forward.

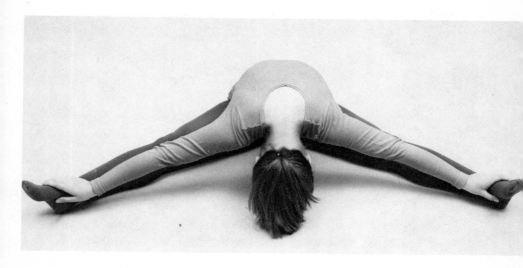

Can you touch the floor with your forehead?

to press your face to your knees. Remain in the pose for about five breaths, trying to press closer each time you exhale.

Variation 2. Spread your legs as far apart as you can, after you have reached the sitting position, and try to press your head to the floor between them. Stretch your arms out along the length of your legs and try to reach your big toes. Alternately, you can clasp your hands behind your head and push it gently toward the floor. Hold the pose for five breaths, pressing down as you exhale. Toes in this position should be turned slightly inward to give a "pigeon-toed" effect.

The Locust

Until the muscles in your back have grown stronger, you should build up to the Full Locust by doing the Half Locust at least ten times a day. Even if you are perfectly capable of doing the Full Locust, it's a good idea to go through two Half Locusts first. This is simply a precaution against pulling a back muscle.

The Half Locust

1. Lie face down on the floor with the soles of your feet turned up. Raise you head enough to place your chin on the floor and push it forward as far as you can. Your arms should lie alongside your body, palms down.

2. Slowly lift your left leg as high as you can without bending your knee. Don't tense your calf or point your toes. And don't cheat by tilting your pelvis. The muscle in the small of your back should be doing the work. This is a Half Locust.

3. Pause for a moment with your leg in the air, then lower it carefully to the floor and repeat with your right leg.

The Full Locust

1. Lie as before, but this time clench your fists to provide more strength. Your thumbs can be up or point toward the floor,

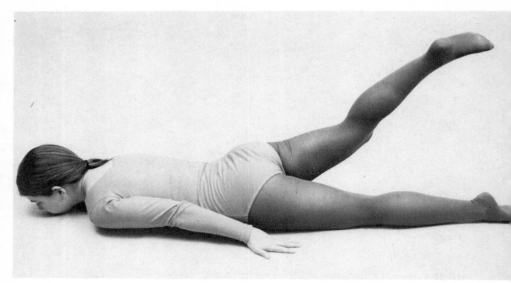

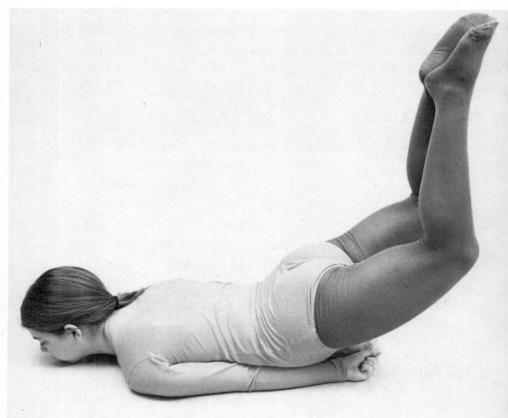

depending on which is more comfortable for you. Try to keep your shoulders on or near the floor during the Full Locust.

2. Keeping your feet together and your knees straight, raise both legs and hips as high as you can, pushing with your fists and chin. Again, be careful not to point your toes or tense your calves.

3. Try to hold your feet in the air for a few seconds before lowering them. If you can't do that at first, at least don't let them drop, but bring them down in a controlled way. Keep your breathing as normal as you can. This is more difficult than in most of the exercises, but it is important. If you catch yourself holding your breath, try again.

Incidentally, the Locust Pose, which is obviously useful in strengthening your back muscles, is also marvellously effective for people with chronic backache. If you have any problems that way — and teenagers do as well as old people — work hard on your Locust.

The Half Locust is fairly easy . . .
. . . the Full Locust is difficult!

The Bow

Like the Cobra Pose (which you assume as part of the Salute
to the Sun, but which can also be done as a separate pose) and
the Locust, the Bow is a backward bending exercise. It combines
elements of the other two, and for some people it's more difficult than either. The thing to remember is to go at it smoothly
and easily without attempting to force anything. This warning
goes with all yoga exercises, of course, but for good measure
gets repeated before the ones in which you might be especially
tempted to forget it.

1. Lie down on your stomach and, bending your knees backward, reach back to grasp your ankles with your hands. Do this
so that the palms of your hands are on the outsides of the ankles
with fingers reaching around the front. Your thumb should also
be in line with your fingers, not hooked underneath. This grip is
important, so check with the picture to make sure you have it
right. Your knees should be slightly apart, but your toes should
touch. Your chin is raised slightly from the floor.

2. Now push your feet back and up, keeping your toes together. Your hips will rise from the floor as your back arches,
till you are, in effect, balanced on your stomach. As your thigh
muscles — which are doing the work — grow stronger, you'll
be able to arch till your knees are higher than your head.

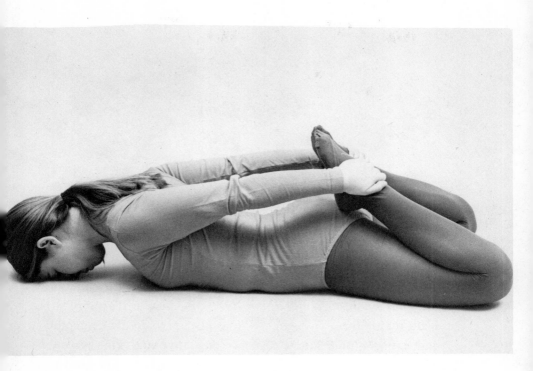

The start of the Bow.

3. As soon as you reach the preceding position, begin to *rock* forward and backward. At first you will only rock back and forth on your stomach, but eventually you can really get some action going, rocking back and forth from your chest to your thighs. Don't push it. Be careful to keep your arms straight and completely relaxed — there's a tendency to tense them. It's impossible to relax your back completely, but don't tense it either. Rock *smoothly,* not jerkily. The best way to breathe is to inhale as your head goes up and exhale as it goes down. Definitely don't hold your breath.

4. Stop rocking slowly and hold the pose at the starting position for a moment before returning slowly to the floor.

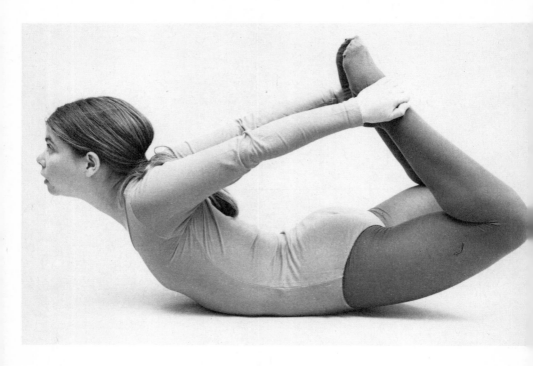

Try rocking back and forth like this.

The Bow is hard on almost anyone's thigh muscles at first, but the pain will pass as they grow stronger. This is one of the exercises that is particularly good for people who are somewhat overweight, though it's also harder on them! Flabby muscles in the stomach and thighs get a marvellous workout, and if you have any problems in those areas, you should be able to see improvement literally within a week. And you'll be able to *feel* something in a single day — that is an unconditional guarantee!

The Triangle

You've been bending your spine backward and forward in truly amazing fashion in the previous exercises, but don't think that yoga neglects the *sides* of your torso. This *asana* and the following one make sure that you will eventually be able to twist yourself in any direction at all.

1. Stand up on your mat, placing your feet two or three feet apart with the toes pointed comfortably out. Raise your arms at the sides to shoulder level, palms down.

2. Slowly bend to your left, being careful to stay in the same plane — that is, don't lean forward or back. Slide your left hand down your leg going as far as you can toward the ankle. Your right arm, meanwhile, comes up so that it's right next to your ear, which causes a good pull on your side muscles, including the area just above your hips.

3. Straighten slowly, and from the standing position, repeat the exercise to the right. Do the whole thing four times, and be sure to do it the yogic way — not in a vigorous Western "up-down, up-down" way.

4. From the standing position, twist your body so that you're looking over your right shoulder. Now bend down and touch your right foot with your left hand, looking backward the whole time.

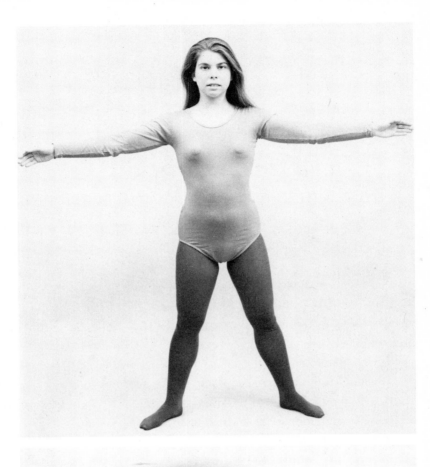

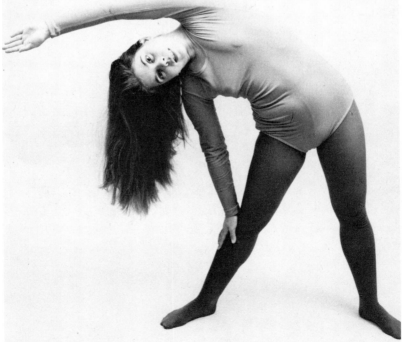

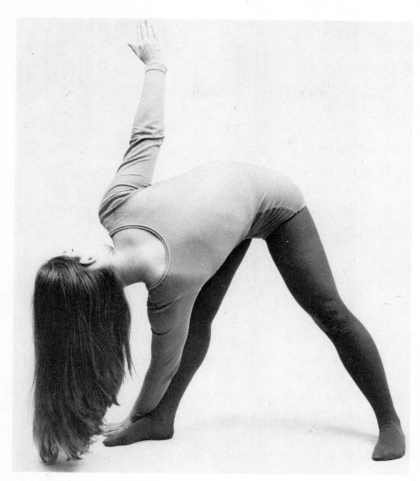

Look over your shoulder as you bend.

5. Straighten slowly, and reverse the procedure, this time touching your left foot with your right hand.

Errors to avoid in the triangle pose are bending your knees, leaning slightly forward in the first variation, and not looking backward in the second. When you're doing everything right, you should be able to feel a long pull right down the sides of your body. Don't worry if you can't reach your ankle or your foot. You'll stretch soon enough.

Top: raise your arms to shoulder level.
Bottom: keep your body on the same plane.

The Twist

Some people, if you tell them you're studying yoga, will say, "Oh, you mean where you twist yourself up into a pretzel!" What you usually do then is grunt or mumble something in a disgusted tone, because really that is not what yoga is all about. Nevertheless, some yogic *asanas* do have their pretzel-like aspects. To do most of them, you have to be fairly advanced, but for this Twist you simply have to be limber.

Actually, the Twist is rather marvellous looking when you finally get it all together. It is a completely static pose, so you don't have to do anything once you do get there, just sit and look elegant and push gently. Getting there is, however, difficult to describe, so follow the directions carefully and study the pictures before you start. It is not as hard to do as it is to explain.

1. Sit on the floor and tuck your right heel into your crotch.

2. Place your left foot alongside your right knee on the outside of the leg. Your left anklebone should be closer to you than the right knee, but the end of your foot protrudes beyond it.

3. With your right hand reach down to grasp your left instep. Do this so that your elbow is on the outside of the standing knee, pressing against it. Keep your right knee pressed to the floor.

One foot at your crotch, the other at your knee.

38

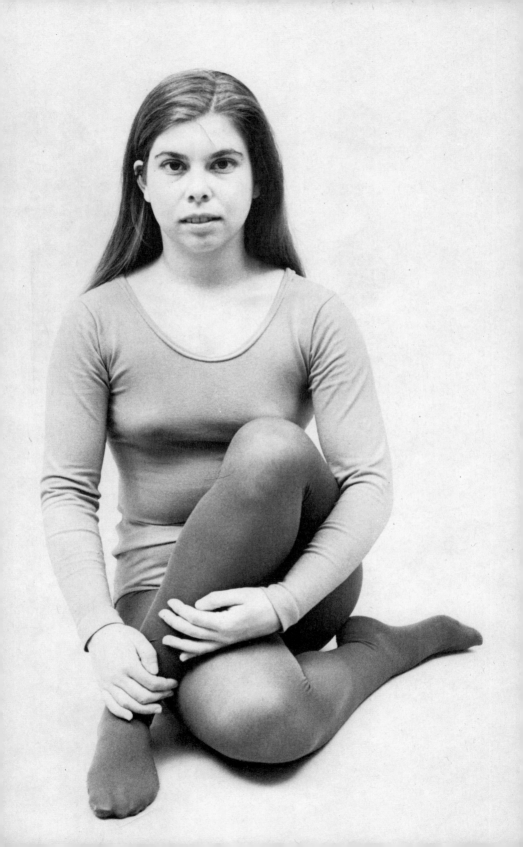

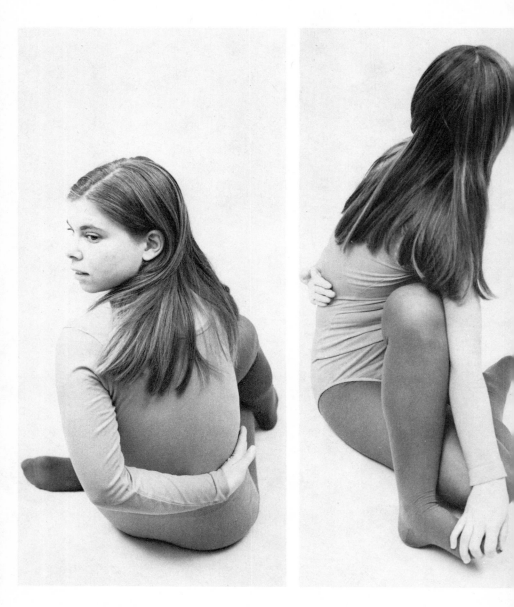

Left: try to reach right around your back.
Right: grasp your foot as your elbow presses your knee.

40

4. With your left hand, reach around your back and try to touch your right thigh. Use your right arm as a lever working on the fulcrum of your left knee to twist you further. Make sure you're sitting on *both* buttocks. Sit very straight, with your chin held high.

5. Turn your head to look behind you, as far as it will go. Look noble; it is the only possible expression for this position. Hold this position, continuing to gently press the body further in the twist and keeping your spine relaxed. Breathe evenly and deeply about five times.

6. Come back to a normal sitting position slowly, and now reverse the pose, starting by folding your left leg.

Older people sometimes have difficulty with this pose, but there's really no reason why you should unless you're carrying a fair amount of extra weight. If you do find it too hard, try it with the folded leg (that's the right leg in the order described above) stretched out in front instead. If you do that, use your left hand as a prop to lean on instead of trying to reach around your back with it.

The
Headstand

People who don't know yoga from yogurt and don't care can
get excited about the Headstand. For some reason they really like
to watch someone stand on his head. Maybe it's the kid in them
coming out — most little kids try to stand on their heads and
some of them get pretty good at it. Any *big* kid who tried to
learn to stand on his head in the slaphappy way little ones do
could get hurt, however. In the first place, little kids are made
of india rubber. And again, you know the old saying, "the bigger
they are the harder they fall."

In yoga it's considered folly to try to do a headstand all at
once without first strengthening your neck. If you studied with
a master yogi, you might have to do your preliminary exercise
for a month before he permitted you to let your feet rise from
the floor, and even after that he might not let you straighten your
legs upward for another week. No master yogi is watching over
you now, but you can and should monitor yourself. Do steps
1 through 6 for at least a week (longer if you feel at all dizzy
or insecure) before you lift your feet from the ground. Then,
when you do lift them, don't attempt to straighten your knees
till you are quite comfortably secure and in no danger of col-
lapsing. Patience is important in yoga, and the headstand is
where you should start practicing it.

In the section on the Salute to the Sun, I suggested that if you spend your first sessions learning to relax and next the several steps to the Salute, you might follow with the initial stages of the Headstand. This is an intelligent way to go about your yoga routine, starting each day with what you have already learned and then adding one or at the most two new exercises a day. If you do that, by the time you actually get to the Headstand you'll be ready to go up in the air. If you learn the poses in order you will actually save time and quell your impatience. More about this later.

1. Fold your towel in two and kneel on it. It might be more comfortable to work on a rug, even if you don't use one for the other poses.

2. Lock your fingers together and place them on the towel in such a way that your head can rest against your fingers to form one base of an equilateral triangle with your elbows as the other two bases.

3. Lean your head lightly against your fingers, placing it so that the weight rests approximately midway between the crown and the forehead. You will determine this point quite naturally as you continue to work on the initial steps day by day. You will also learn to determine the proper angle of your elbows.

4. Straighten your legs, leaning on your toes and taking some weight on your head.

5. Now begin to walk toward your head slowly, taking tiny steps. Let your weight rest on your head rather than your arms. When you get so close to the body that your legs rise involuntarily, stop. Just stay there for a moment or two, getting used to the situation.

6. Slowly walk backward till your feet are where they were. Then go down to your knees and elbows and lift your head as you did in the beginning position. Roll your head around on your neck a few times, then repeat the whole procedure at least

43

twice, holding it a little longer at the point where you begin to rise each time.

7. After a week or so of doing the above preliminary exercises faithfully, you're ready to go up, but not too far up. This time, let your legs rise, keeping your knees bent and your feet against your thighs. Stay in that position as long as you feel comfortable, which will probably be only a few seconds. Relax your muscles and try to determine if the nape of your neck is positioned properly. If you do fall, you will collapse forward, so there is no need to have a wall behind you. Come down from this position gently, on your toes, and walk back to the starting position.

8. When you are *quite secure* with your legs bent — which should take a few days — you can proceed to the next step, which is to point your knees to the ceiling, keeping your feet against your thighs. If you feel at all unsteady, don't go further than this, but simply hold this position as long as you can and then go down the way you came.

9. When your knees are pointed upward, you can then raise your feet. Adjust yourself carefully to maintain balance. Don't try to stay up more than a few seconds at first, and when you come down, do it slowly and gracefully, retracing your steps in reverse. Rest in the kneeling position a few moments.

An important point to remember while standing on your head is to breathe through your nose. Some people have trouble doing this, but they must discipline themselves.

Quite ordinary people in India take great pride in the fact that they do the Headstand every morning, bragging about how long they stay up, especially if it's more than fifteen minutes.

Top: your hands and elbows form a triangle.
Bottom: walk right up toward your head.

44

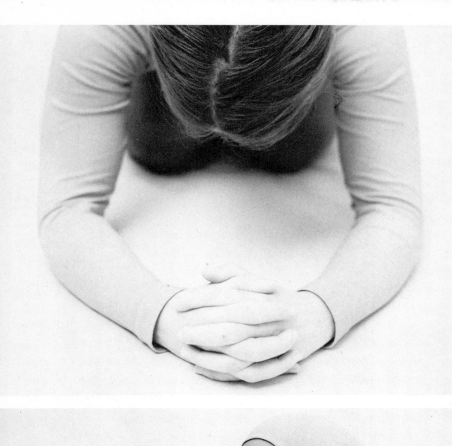
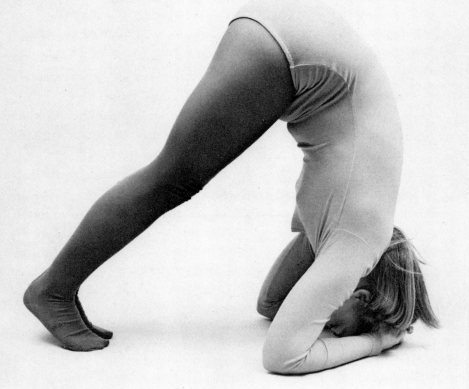

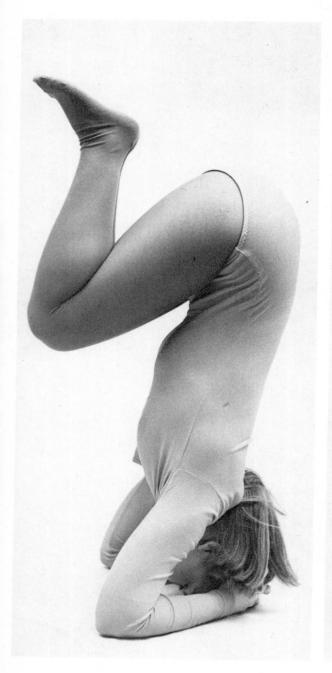
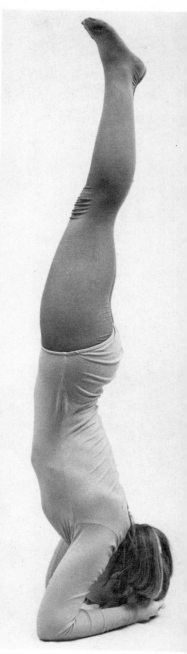

46

You can stay up that long too, if you really want to. But don't rush it — the people who are bragging have been at it for years.

After you get good at the Headstand, you can start having a little fun with it. You can bring your legs down to the floor one at a time, spread them wide, or twist them around each other. You can do the Lotus position standing on your head too, but you'd better not try it till you can sit in the Lotus the ordinary way first.

To hear some people tell it, the Headstand is like old-fashioned snake oil medicine: good for just about everything that ails you. They say it benefits the bones, the blood, the brain, the lungs, the innards, and the tired feet, not to mention skin, hair, eyes, ears, nose, and throat. Who knows? Perhaps it's all true. If you want to find out, just keep standing on your head, and after ten years or so, compare yourself to people who don't. The odds are in your favor.

Left: keep your knees bent as you rise.
Right: the Headstand.

The Lotus

The Lotus Pose and its easier variations, the Easy Pose and the Adept's Pose, are known as "meditative poses." Rather than being an end in itself, each of these poses is intended to be an adjunct to breathing exercises and to meditation. To sit in one position for a long time, motionless, with a straight spine is considered essential to concentration.

Few of us are able to do the Lotus at first; it is especially difficult for boys. You should work up to it gradually, using the Adept's Pose at first for your breathing exercises, or, if that is too uncomfortable, the Easy Pose. Exercise the legs and feet till you are able to take the Lotus, if only for a few seconds at first. In any group of ten people, each will be at a different level of agility and some really can't manage anything other than the Easy Pose at first.

The Easy Pose

This is simply an ordinary cross-legged position on the floor. Be sure to sit erect with your back straight. Put one hand on each knee and push slowly and steadily toward the floor. Do this five times every day, and you'll soon be ready for the next stage.

The Easy Pose.

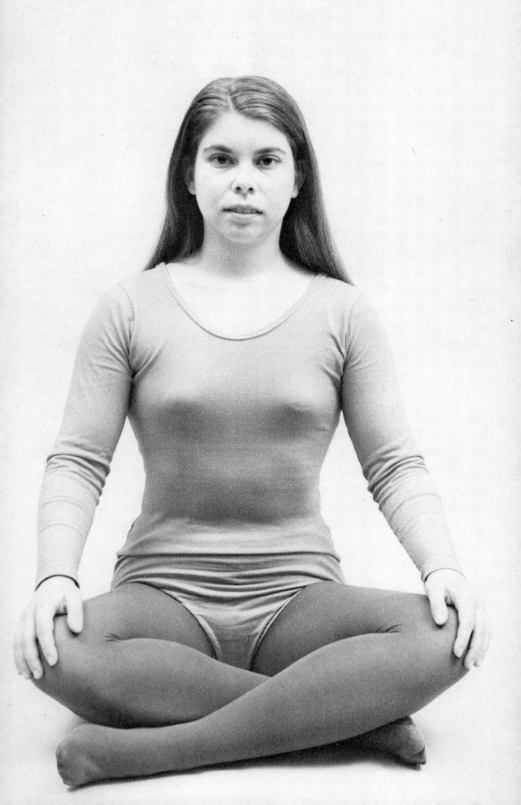

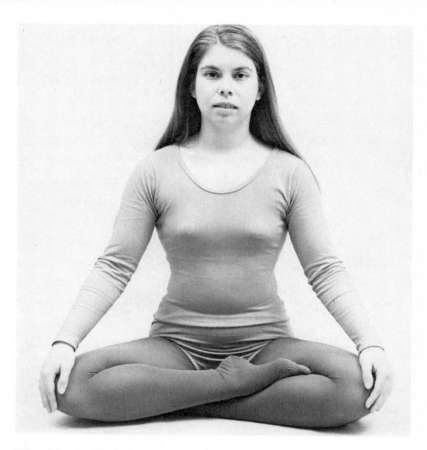

The Adept's Pose.

The Adept's Pose

Fold your left leg so that the heel fits snugly against your crotch. Then fold your right leg and place the foot over the left so that your right heel rests against your pubic bone. Sit very erect. If this pose is easier for you with the legs reversed, that is, with the right leg under the left, by all means do it that way.

The Lotus

Most people need practice getting into the Lotus Pose.

1. Sit erect with your feet stretched out in front of you. Then fold your left knee, heel against your crotch. Take your right

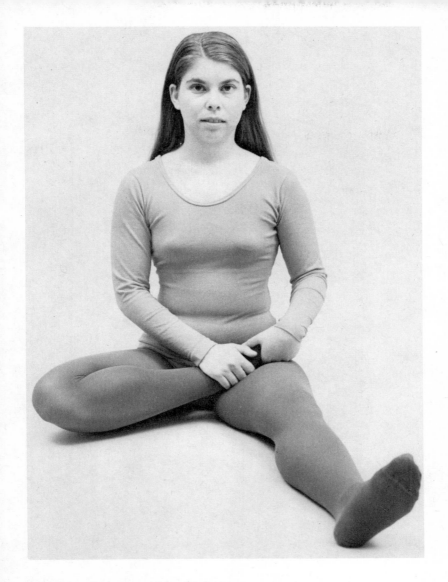

Bring one leg up to your thigh.

foot with both hands and place it on your left thigh, bringing the right heel as close as possible to your stomach. Straighten the right leg out and repeat about ten times.

2. Reverse the position, folding the right leg and bringing in the left.

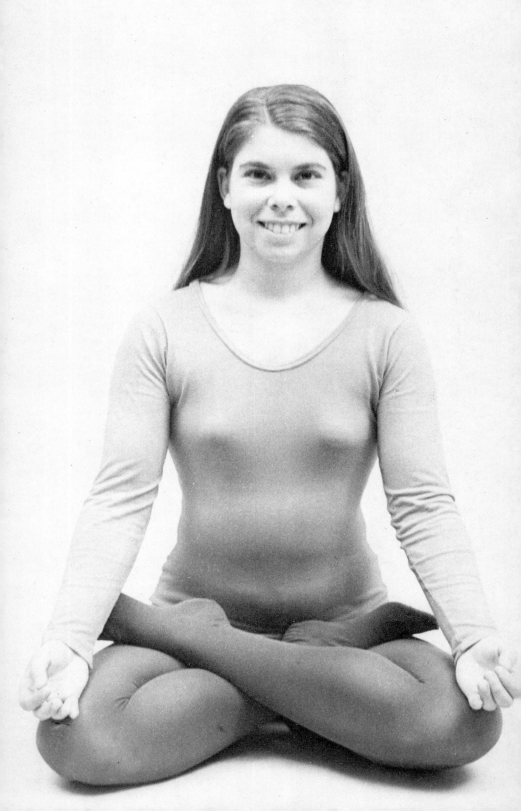

3. For the Lotus proper, place your right foot on your left thigh first, as above. Then pull your left foot in and place it on your right thigh. Hold the position as long as you can, breathing evenly. You will find yourself sitting very erect. When you come out of the Lotus, do so slowly. Shake your legs up afterward to get any "kinks" out.

Your Hands

As you see in the pictures, hands in the meditative positions are held in *padmasan*. The thumb forms a circle with the index finger, and the other fingers form a relaxed half-curve. The hands are then rested lightly on the knees. This is a most comfortable way of placing the hands and stops any impulse you may have toward nervous fidgeting.

In the following breathing exercises, sit in whichever position you can most comfortably manage, though eventually you will want to use the Lotus. The upper body should be relaxed but very erect. You should be able to hold the same position throughout the breathing exercises, but don't be annoyed with yourself if you can't. In yoga, the emphasis is on *slow* mastery of the body.

The Lotus — note hand position.

Breathing

Chances are you haven't spent a major part of your life thinking about breathing. If you weren't already an expert breather, you wouldn't be here to read the page. Yet there's a world of difference between proper and improper breathing. Yoga teaches that breathing correctly is absolutely essential to good health and a sense of well-being. In addition, experts in yoga gain great control and mastery over their breathing. This takes many years to learn, but the kind of breathing you, as a beginner, should learn is very easy once you get the knack of it.

You must first learn to isolate the three separate breathing areas. The best way is to get a belt with notches or buckle holes in it, and then to lie down flat on your back.

First, buckle the belt around the lower part of your ribs, well above your waist. Now exhale all the air you possibly can.

Imagine that you are a kind of balloon with a long hose reaching from your nose right down to your abdomen. Imagine that any air coming through the hose has to fill you from the bottom up. Now inhale slowly, letting your abdominal area expand naturally and swell with the air. If your chest starts to get into the act, the belt will restrain it. Breathe in and out from this region only till you get the hang of it. This is called *diaphragmatic* breathing. It's considered the best kind. Actors, sing-

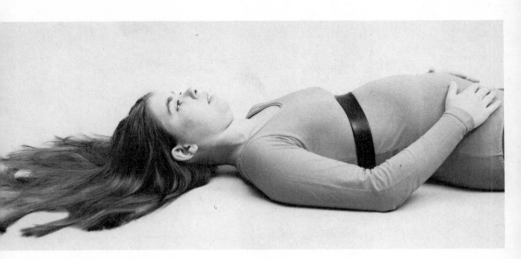

Breathing with the abdomen.

ers, swimmers, and others practice it especially. For some reason, it comes much more naturally to men than to women.

2. Unbuckle the belt and now cinch it around your waist or abdomen. Exhale completely, and keep your stomach muscles taut so you won't breathe from the diaphragm. Hold the sides of your rib cage with your hands. Now breathe in, expanding your ribs and trying to push your hands even farther apart. You'll notice that you have to use more effort to get a good breath this way. Breathe in and out till you've worked out just how this kind of breathing — *chest* breathing — differs from the diaphragmatic type.

3. Now try to immobilize both your chest and your stomach and, after exhaling, breathe by drawing your collarbone up toward your chin (this sounds impossible, but it's actually the way quite a few people, mostly women, breathe). By itself, this method is most wasteful and inefficient, but when it's integrated into complete breathing, it becomes useful. You don't have to practice this kind of breathing after you've learned how to do it.

55

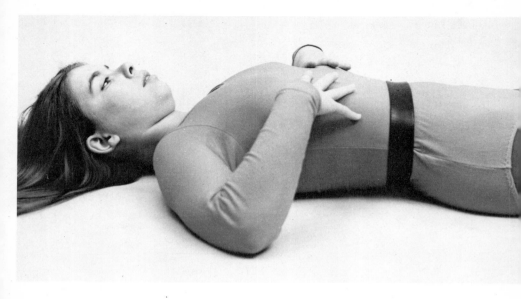

Breathing with the chest.

After you've removed the belt, practice complete breathing, still lying on your back. Use the analogy of the balloon with the hose again. This time, let your stomach fill with air, as you did before, but now, when it is full, expand your ribs and let your chest fill too. Don't jerk your action, it should be continuous. Also don't draw in your stomach muscles as you expand your chest. When your chest is full, raise your collarbone slightly to let in a little more air. Do this several times, using the technique you have learned. Now begin to concentrate on the ratio of inhalation to exhalation. It should be 1:2 — that is, a breath should take twice as long to leave your body as to enter it. This does not come absolutely naturally, but is not hard so long as you don't breathe in for too long a count at first. Start with four seconds in and eight seconds out. Gradually, you can increase the number of seconds, but keep the ratio the same.

Practice this kind of breathing until it has become second

nature to you. You don't have to confine it simply to your lessons; you can do a spot of yogic breathing anywhere — in a classroom, on the bus, in bed. When you no longer have trouble timing your exhalations properly, the next step is to hold your breath. The ratio now becomes 1:4:2 — that is, you hold your breath for four times as long as you breathe in and twice as long as you breathe out. Start with four seconds again, then hold it for sixteen, and exhale for eight. Take your time in increasing this to a longer count. As with everything else in yoga, breathing should be done in a relaxed way.

Your Routine

Along the way, remarks have been made about the order of the exercises, but it's a good idea to get everything straight about this in one place. The exercises contained in this book are very basic, and you are intended to do them all, in the order set forth, every day. Once you become skilled at them, the whole sequence should take about half an hour.

The reason you should do them in order is practical, not mystical. Forward bending exercises are balanced with backward bending ones. Under different teachers, the order varies a little — for instance, the Headstand may be done earlier or the Shoulder Stand later. Here they are placed at the beginning and end of the sequence so as to separate the inverted postures.

When you are first learning yoga, however, it's not a good idea to try to do all the poses at once. Instead, tackle them one at a time, adding a new one only when you are really certain of your skill with the previous one. Again you should proceed in order, with certain exceptions which are listed here.

1. As was suggested in the section on the Salute to the Sun, if it takes you a long time to perfect this fairly active exercise, you might not attempt to go farther for a while. Instead, you can follow up with the preliminary steps to the Headstand, following that with breathing exercises — the early ones where you are lying on the floor.

58

2. Always begin and end with relaxation. Don't skimp on this; it's very good for your body. You may want to do your end relaxation after the Headstand and before you begin your breathing.

3. After you have mastered all the exercises and have made them into a daily habit, if you are ever pressed for time, you can eliminate some of them judiciously. You might restrict yourself to one forward bending exercise and one backward bending one and eliminate the Twist and the Headstand. You should try not to skip too often, however, as none of these *asanas* duplicates another. Each calls distinctly different muscles into play.

4. If you can really only manage a mini-session, do the Salute to the Sun and the Shoulder–Stand–Plow, relax briefly and try to fit your breathing in during some odd moments later.

Some people like to do the Salute all by itself in the morning as a wake-up tonic, and then repeat it later in the day at the start of their regular session. It's a splendid way to start the day, and if you wanted to, you could combine it with another exercise, like the Triangle. Don't forget that you are doing yoga, not calisthenics — maintain that smooth easy rhythm.

Further Study

If you get interested in yoga, you will eventually want to study with a teacher. As a matter of fact, you really have to study with someone at least for a while, because the movements in a yogic *asana* are so precise and you must make certain to do them correctly. A teacher will be able to see what you are doing right or wrong far better than you can yourself.

Fortunately, finding a teacher has become easy. Small towns often have someone giving yoga classes. Big cities have dozens of them. What's more, yoga teachers usually don't charge much, although you can't count on that absolutely.

This book was designed for you to use at home, though there's no reason why you couldn't use it as a supplemental handbook while studying in a class. If you are careful as you learn the different positions there's no way you can harm yourself. You'll find your body becoming more supple and malleable in a matter of days; things you thought were impossible will become increasingly probable. Touching your head to your knees, for instance — you may not be able to do it yet, but at least you're willing to consider the notion of one day achieving it.

Some classes and some other books go into questions of religion and diet and so forth which you won't find here. You don't have to make yoga a whole way of life to derive benefits from it.

The vast majority of people in both the East and the West who practice yoga habitually do so for its physical benefits and because it helps their concentration. That's the approach we've taken here.

You know by this time that yoga is fun. It really is a tremendous source of satisfaction, all the more so as it is completely noncompetitive. You're working with and against your own body, and as your body gets into better and better shape, working with and against it becomes even more fun.

Index

63